The liver diseases antidote:

making your liver fit and disease-free

By

Anthony S. Macklin

Disclaimer

All rights reserved.

No portion of this book may be reproduced in any form without written permission from the publisher or author, except as permitted by U.S. copyright law.

Concerning the topic matter covered, this publication is intended to offer reliable information. It is offered for sale with the knowledge that neither the author nor the book's publisher is involved in providing accounting, legal, or other professional services. Despite the publisher's and author's best efforts in the preparation of this book, they expressly disclaim any implied guarantees of fitness or merchantability for a specific purpose and make no promises or warranties regarding the correctness or completeness of its contents. Sales representatives and written sales materials are not authorized to establish or extend any warranties. The suggestions and tactics offered here might not be appropriate for your circumstance. When necessary, you should seek expert advice.

Table of contents

Disclaimer

Table of contents

Introduction

Chapter 1

The illness of the liver

What exactly is the liver?

Chapter 2

Causes of liver diseases

Chapter 3

Symptoms of liver diseases

Chapter 4

Diagnosis and management

Conclusion

Introduction

Today, millions of Americans suffer from chronic illnesses such as cardiovascular disease, diabetes, and gastrointestinal disorders. Despite recent developments in modern medicine in the past few years, chronic illness has remained a mystery to physicians. The complete extent of the body's functioning and capabilities has not been discovered by science, and this is especially true for the liver.

People are conscious of the various organs found in their bodies, such as the heart or intestines, yet most are unaware of their livers. They are not required to. The liver's incredible abilities are not easily evident until there is a tremendous breakdown in functioning. Although the liver's importance in sustaining health is often overlooked, it works relentlessly to keep humans healthy.

The liver is responsible for a variety of vital processes. Its primary function is to process lipids and protect the pancreas. The liver can also contain glycogen and glucose, along with a variety of nutrients, minerals, vitamins, and dietary fiber. When certain nutrients are deficient in the food, the liver draws on these reserves. Furthermore, this organ neutralizes harmful toxins and other substances, ensuring that blood is pure before it is pumped to the heart. The liver has it unique immune system that protects it against viruses that endanger overall health. This immune system protects against viruses and other pathogens that are so deep down the surface that medical professionals are oblivious to their presence.

The liver also has an innate intelligence, such as the ability to predict when it might need to create more bilirubin to aid in fat breakdown.

The liver is much more than just an organ. The liver contains vast wisdom that is intimately related to mental, physical, and emotional well-being. Honoring the liver will result in increased inner serenity and well-being, which will emanate out into the larger world.

Cirrhosis of the liver affects individuals between the ages of 40 and 60, and rates among younger people have been rising for several decades. In reality, between 2009 and 2016, mortality from alcohol-related cirrhosis increased by 10% on average among people aged 25 to 34.

Chapter 1

The illness of the liver

What exactly is the liver?

First, we must comprehend the liver's duties, strengths, and weaknesses.

The liver is the body's largest organ for good reason: it carries out over 500 distinct functions. Keeping blood sugar, electrolytes (Sodium, potassium, chloride, etc.), and blood pressure in balance; changing the amino acids to numerous substances and into sugar; fat production and burning; digestion and dispersion of food; metabolism and removal of medicines and compounds are just a few of the functions that the liver performs.

When we eat, fat undergoes digestion with the aid of bile, which the liver produces and releases. This bile is absorbed again into the body after absorption and returns to the liver. More than half of the body's cholesterol is used for making bile.

Sugars and amino acids get absorbed into circulation after carbohydrates and proteins are digested and sent to the liver, which distributes them throughout the body.

The liver is responsible for processing all food and medicine that we ingest. The more medications and food our bodies absorb, the greater the strain on the liver.

What exactly is liver disease?

The notion of "liver disease" applies to any condition affecting the liver. These various liver diseases can develop due to a variety of factors, however, they all possess the possibility which is to injure your liver and slowing down its daily operation.

Liver disease is a typical term frequently used to refer to a variety of conditions that harm or affect the liver. When substances pass through the body's digestive system, the liver's job is to extract nutrients from the waste.

Bile, a fluid produced by the liver, is a chemical that removes poisons from the body. Several liver diseases are caused when the liver fails to perform this job.

Liver disorders require prompt treatment. It needs to be properly diagnosed and treated because, if ignored, it can lead to severe life-threatening problems.

A healthy liver is necessary for supporting several functions, including digestion and detoxification. The liver can be harmed by a poor lifestyle or excessive booze consumption. Cirrhosis, hepatitis, and fatty liver are among the most common liver diseases that require medical care.

Let's take a peek at some of the most common liver diseases.

1. Hepatitis

Hepatitis is a viral illness that causes liver damage. It inflames and damages your liver, rendering it difficult for it to function correctly. Hepatitis is classified into five types: A, B, C, and D. They are entirely distinct viruses and infections.

Hepatitis is a liver inflammation caused by a variety of factors, including viruses or illnesses.

Hepatitis manifests itself in the following ways:

Hepatitis A: Hepatitis A is a virus infection of the liver. It produces a short-term or acute infection. This illness is spread through unsanitary practices and careless food handling. It is also known as viral hepatitis. Hepatitis A is transmitted through the fecal-oral pathway. Hepatitis A is believed to spread primarily through poor hand hygiene and unsanitary conditions.One can completely recover and gain lifelong immunity to Hepatitis A.

Hepatitis B: hepatitis B is an example of viral hepatitis. It can induce a short-term (acute) or long-term (chronic) infection. hepatitis B is spread through blood, sperm, and bodily secretions. It is conceivable for a mother to give birth to her child. Hepatitis B, on the other hand, has a vaccine that is extremely effective at prevention, however, cannot yet be cured in the instance of chronic infection. There are treatments known to delay or stop viral replication and thus limit the progression of the disease in infected people. On treatment, one can heal in 6-7 months and become immune to further hepatitis B infection.

Approximately 80% of individuals with this disease develop a chronic infection. Many individuals with the disease have no symptoms.

Hepatitis C: is spread through blood and physical activity. The main cause of liver disease, cancer, and liver failure is chronic hepatitis C. Antiviral medications can get the infection out of the body. There hepatitis C vaccine is not accessible, and the immunity status is unclear. (for A and B viruses, vaccination is possible.)

2. Fatty liver syndrome

When the liver accumulates too much fat, such as in cases of obesity or type 2 diabetes, the fatty liver disease develops.

Abuse of alcohol increases triglyceride and cholesterol danger. Alcohol abuse is not a factor in the buildup of these chemicals in the liver that results in fatty liver disease. Other terms for fatty liver disease include non-alcoholic steatohepatitis and non-alcoholic fatty liver disease (NAFLD). (NASH).

The fatty liver disease primarily comes in two forms:

i). <u>Alcoholic fatty liver</u> - Alcoholic fatty liver refers to the buildup of fat in the liver as a consequence of heavy drinking.

ii). <u>Non-alcoholic liver disease</u> - Non-alcoholic fatty liver disease affects individuals who do not drink heavily.

3. Autoimmune disorders

In cases where your immune system targets cells that are healthy in your body, autoimmune illnesses develop. Numerous autoimmune conditions exist, including primary biliary cirrhosis and autoimmune hepatitis.

The human body is supported by an immune system that defends against exterior threats like bacteria and viruses. Rarely, for several reasons, the body's immune system will target healthy cells. Attacks on healthy liver cells can cause inflammation and scarring. Examples include viral hepatitis, primary biliary cholangitis (PBC), and primary sclerosing cholangitis (PSC). Instances of autoimmune liver diseases include autoimmune hepatitis.

4. Genetic disorders

Several hereditary conditions that you get from either of your parents can also impact your liver.

5. Cancer

The liver is where liver cancer starts. When cancer starts somewhere else in the body and moves to the liver, it is referred to as secondary liver cancer.

One form of liver cancer is hepatocellular carcinoma.

6. Cirrhosis

The scarring of the liver due to diseases and other liver injuries, such as drinking, is known as cirrhosis. If alcohol is taken frequently, the liver might become nervous. The liver tissues can become stiffer and lose their capacity over time. The damage is regarded as destructive and irreversible due to the chance of liver failure.

Chapter 2

Causes of liver diseases

There are different reasons for liver illness, they are as per the following:

Disease: The liver can become tainted by infections, which brings about irritation and diminished liver capability. The infections that hurt the liver can be sent through blood or semen, debased food or water, or direct contact with a tainted person. Hepatitis infections are the most common reasons of liver disease, the infections include:

Hepatitis A

Hepatitis B

Hepatitis C

After Contaminations the beneath are the significant reasons for liver illness:

1. Sure over-the-counter or professionally prescribed drugs.
2. A couple of natural fixings
3. **Immune system conditions**:

   The liver might be influenced by immune system illnesses, which happen when the insusceptible framework assaults specific body organs. Your invulnerable framework wards off intruders including microorganisms and infections. Yet, it could turn out badly and assault at least one piece of your body, like your liver.

Different immune system liver circumstances include:

Hepatitis auto-immune: inflames your liver. It can prompt different issues and, surprisingly, liver disappointment. It strikes young ladies more frequently than young men.

Essential Biliary cholangitis: assaults little cylinders in your liver called bile pipes. They convey bile, a compound that assists you with processing food. At the point when the pipes are harmed, the bile upholds inside your liver and scars it. Ladies catch this more frequently than men.

First-stage sclerosing cholangitis: scars your bile channels, and it can ultimately hinder them. The bile develops inside your liver, and that makes it harder for your liver to work. It might prompt liver malignant growth, and you could sometimes require a liver transfer. Men are almost more certain than ladies to get it.

4. Hereditary qualities: The development of various destructive substances in the liver can bring about liver problems in the event that you have a broken quality obtained from your folks.

The hereditary hepatic circumstances involve:

Hemochromatosis: makes your body store up a lot of the iron from your food. The additional iron develops in your liver, heart, or different organs. It can prompt perilous circumstances like liver illnesses, coronary illness, or diabetes.

<u>Wilson's illness</u>: makes copper develop in your liver and different organs. Its most memorable side effects as a rule show up when you're between the ages of 6 and 35, most frequently in your teenagers. It influences your liver, however, it can cause nerve and mental issues.

<u>An absence of alpha-1 antitrypsin</u>: involves a substance that assists your lungs with opposing diseases. Your liver makes it. Be that as it may, when your liver misunderstands the recipe, the broken substance can develop and cause liver sickness.

5. Malignant development:

The disease appears in your liver, which is probably because it has spread from one more piece of your body, similar to your lungs, colon, or bosom.

Be that as it may, a couple of tumors can begin in the liver.

<u>Liver tumor</u>: affects ladies more frequently than men, and African-Americans more frequently than whites. Your PCP could call it hepatocellular carcinoma. It's more probable assuming you have hepatitis or drink excessively.

<u>Liver cell adenoma</u> is a growth that doesn't have a disease. It's phenomenal, however, ladies who take conception prevention pills for quite a while are more inclined than others to foster it.

There's little opportunity for the growth that could ultimately transform into disease.

Biliary duct cancer: The bile ducts, which transport the fluid that aids in food digestion from your liver to your small intestine, are attacked by biliary duct cancer. This type of cancer is uncommon and primarily affects individuals over 50.

6. Development of fat in the liver (nonalcoholic greasy liver illness)

is when an excessive amount of fat has developed inside your liver. The additional fat hcan excite your liver. One kind of NAFLD is nonalcoholic steatohepatitis (NASH). It implies you have irritation and cell harm in your liver, as well as fat. It can scar your liver and lead to different problems, similar to cirrhosis.

7. A Non-cancerous growth is a liver cell adenoma. Although it's rare, long-term birth control pill users are more likely than other people to acquire it. There is a slight possibility that the tumor will ultimately develop into cancer.

8. Chronic drinking

In addition to alcohol, your liver is a strong organ that can process many other toxic substances, either making them harmless or even recovering some nutritional value from them. There is a cap, though, and if you go over it every day, that's all there is to it.

The liver converts alcohol into simple sugars after a series of steps that entail reducing it down into smaller compounds. But some of these intermediary substances are much more harmful than alcohol. They only persist for a brief period before changing into another shape, but they still cause harm.

Currently, your liver can only handle about 30 ml of pure alcohol per hour. If there's more than that, it just continues passing through the liver on each journey until there's a capacity to process it.

However, if you continue to apply pressure, the liver tissue ultimately completely degrades as a result of the toxic effects, which, because the liver attempts to shield you from the harmful effects, are largely restricted to the liver and are amplified by the means of breaking it down. The liver tissue decomposes and transforms into fat.

Risk elements

You may be more vulnerable to developing liver illness if you have:

- Obesity
- diabetes type 2
- Body art or implants
- drug injection with common needles
- Transfusion of blood
- exposure to bodily secretions and blood of others
- Unrestricted intimacy
- exposure to specific toxins or substances
- an inheritance of liver illness

Chapter 3

Symptoms of liver diseases

The majority of the time, liver diseases do not exhibit obvious, distinct signs and symptoms until it is too late. However, some of the common signs and symptoms include:

- Skin and eyes that look yellow (Jaundice)
- nausea and diarrhea
- reduced hunger
- the propensity for bruising readily
- feeling perpetually exhausted and feeble
- stomach ache and bloating
- edema in the ankles and thighs
- Skin itch
- Urine with a dark color

- Pale stool hue
- Continual exhaustion

What other conditions and signs are associated with liver issues?

Several other illnesses and symptoms, such as the following, can be caused by liver issues:

Cirrhosis: Cirrhosis, which is defined by liver scarring and stiffening, can result from chronic liver damage.

Hepatic encephalopathy: Confusion and drowsiness among other symptoms, can result from hepatic encephalopathy, a condition that can happen when the liver fails to remove toxic chemicals from the blood.

Ascites is the term used to describe the accumulation of fluid in the belly that can be brought on by cirrhosis.

Variceal bleeding can expand and weaken the veins in the esophagus and stomach, which can result in variceal bleeding.

Jaundice is a skin and eye yellowing that can happen as a consequence of liver damage.

Weakness and fatigue: Since the liver plays a role in generating energy, liver issues can cause these symptoms.

Vomiting and sickness: are sometimes caused by liver issues because the liver regulates the digestive system.

Itching: Bile buildup in the skin as a result of chronic liver illness can cause itching.

Bruising and easy bleeding: Since the liver contributes to the production and control of blood-clotting factors, liver issues can result in bruising and easy bleeding.

Please get medical help if you encounter any liver-related symptoms. More severe complications can be avoided with early diagnosis and treatment.

Chapter 4

Diagnosis and management

How is hepatic illness identified?

The following procedures to evaluate liver function could be performed on you:

- thorough blood test
- thrombin interval
- studies for liver function
- amount of blood albumin

Your doctor may also suggest one or more tests to correctly identify and determine the cause of liver disease. These may consist of:

- Liver enzyme levels are measured by blood examinations using liver enzymes.

- The international standard ratio, a blood-clotting measurement, is one of the additional evaluations of liver function. (INR). Unusual amounts could be a sign that your liver isn't working properly.

- Imaging tests: Your doctor may use an ultrasound, MRI, or CT scan to check your liver for indications of injury, scarring, or tumors. The degree of liver fat deposition and scarring can be assessed using the fibroid scan, a different specialist form of ultrasound.

- Liver biopsy: A tiny sample of liver tissue is taken during a liver biopsy by your doctor using a fine needle. To search for indicators of liver illness, they examine the tissue.

How is cirrhosis of the liver managed?

Treatment

Your prognosis will determine how to treat your liver condition. In most cases, as part of a medical program that involves careful monitoring of liver function, some liver issues can be treated with lifestyle changes, such as quitting drinking or losing weight. Other liver issues might need surgery or medical intervention to be resolved.

A liver transplant may eventually be necessary for the treatment of liver disease that results in or has already caused liver failure.

Diet

Eat a decent eating routine: Select food sources from all nutrition classes: Grains, organic products, vegetables, meat and beans, milk, and oil. Eat food with fiber: Fiber helps your liver work at an ideal level. Natural products, vegetables, entire grain bread, rice, and oats can deal with your body's fiber needs

Consume a healthy diet

Foods from all dietary groups should be chosen, including grains, fruits, vegetables, meat and beans, milk, and oil. Your liver operates best when you consume fiber. Your body can get all the fiber it requires from fruits, vegetables, whole grains, bread, rice, and cereals.

Healthy living and home remedies

You can frequently improve your liver health by changing certain lifestyle behaviors.

Keep away from red meat, trans fats, handled sugars, and food sources with high-fructose corn syrup.

If you have been given a liver disease diagnosis, your specialist might advise you to:

- Drink alcohol sparingly, if by any means.

- Red meat, trans fats, refined carbohydrates, and meals containing high-fructose corn syrup should all be avoided.

- Exercise with a moderate effort for 30 to 60 minutes three to four times per week.

- If you are overweight, reduce your daily calorie intake by 500 to 1,000 calories.

Elective medication

There is no alternative medicine treatment for the liver illness that has been proven effective. Although some studies have suggested potential advantages, more study is required.

However, some nutritional and herbal supplements can be detrimental to your liver. Liver harm has been linked to more than a thousand prescription drugs and herbal remedies. including:

Germander ma-huang Vitamin A, alerian, mistletoe, skullcap, chaparral, comfrey, kava, and pennyroyal oil.

Before using any complementary or alternative medicines, it's essential to discuss the possible risks with your doctor in order to protect your liver.

It is important to address the underlying cause of early liver cirrhosis to lessen liver damage. The following are the options:

Alcoholic abuse treatment. People who have developed liver disease as a result of binge drinking should make an effort to cut back. A Therapy program for inebriation may be recommended by your doctor if quitting drinking is difficult. It is imperative to refrain from imbibing if you have liver cirrhosis because alcohol in any amount can cause liver cyanosis.

Loss of weight. If they lose weight and control their blood sugar levels, people who have nonalcoholic liver disease and liver "disease" may become healthy.

Drugs to control infectious illnesses. Through targeted therapy of those viruses, medications may be able to reduce any harm to liver cells caused by serum hepatitis or hepatitis C.

Medications to control the various reasons and signs of liver cirrhosis. Certain types of liver cirrhosis may proceed more slowly with medication. Medication may significantly slow the development of primary biliary cirrhosis of the liver in people who have it identified early.

What actions can be taken to stop the onset or progression of liver disease?

Steps to Prevent Liver Disease

- Eat a balanced, low-fat, low-sugar, low-salt diet that is rich in fiber to maintain a healthy diet.

- Regular exercise can lower your risk of developing liver disease and help you keep a healthy weight. Exercise has been shown to lower the chance of liver disease and encourage a healthy liver, but it's crucial to consult a healthcare professional before beginning any new exercise program if you already have a liver condition.

Exercises that improve insulin sensitivity, lower fat storage, and boost blood flow are the best for liver health. This covers exercises like cycling, swimming, and brisk strolling.

- Alcohol should be avoided or consumed in moderation because it increases the chance of liver disease.

- Invest in a vaccine: They can shield you from viral illnesses that can harm your liver.

- Avoid exposure to toxins: Keep your distance from substances that can damage your liver, such as chemicals, pesticides, and more.

- Treat any underlying medical problems that may exist: Liver disease risk can be increased by long-term conditions like obesity, diabetes, and elevated blood pressure.

- Test yourself: Regular liver function tests can aid in the early detection and monitoring of liver illness.

- Quit smoking; smoking has been linked to severe health issues, such as liver disease.

Which diet should be maintained after liver disease is treated?

- You're not required to diet. Consume balanced diet meals and take your medicine.

- A wide range of meals. fruits and veggies in abundance. Just enough salt.

- Since your jaundice has cleared up, you should be cautious when eating fats and progressively increase the amount in your daily diet until you are certain that the fat you consume is not harming you.

- Given that they are much more familiar with your circumstances, you might first want to ask your doctor for advice on a diet.

Conclusion

Millions of people around the world are affected by liver disease, which is a severe and possibly fatal condition. There is no one-size-fits-all cure for fatty liver disease, but there are things you can do to manage the condition and enhance your quality of life. To protect your liver and lower your risk of getting the liver disease, adopt a healthy lifestyle.

You should seek medical help if you exhibit any liver disease signs and be on the lookout for any risk factors that could increase your likelihood of getting the condition.

www.ingramcontent.com/pod-product-compliance
Lightning Source LLC
Chambersburg PA
CBHW061607250726
48657CB00017B/2230